A Fast Food Guide:
How to Eat Right on Date Night

Phillip Despain CFT

Dedicated to my loving wife. Thank you so much for all the love and support. Thank you for putting up with the long hours. I love you.

Dedicated to my kids; don't be afraid to chase your dreams.

I also want to dedicate this book to all those who are trying to make a change a healthy lifestyle. I admire your determination and courage. I hope this book make your journey a little easier.

Table of Contents

Introduction

Changing your lifestyle to a healthier one is not the easiest thing in the world. It's hard to stick to your goals when friends and family are wanting to go out all of the time.

Your goals are difficult enough without having to tell everyone no when they ask you to go out just because you don't know what to eat at the restaurant.

Well now you don't have to! I have personally gone through each of these menus and recommended items that should not hinder your goals in anyway.

This doesn't mean you should live at these restaurants. Cooking at home where you are in complete control is always going to be king. However this book should help make your journey a little easier.

Here is to your goals, your courage and your journey.

Best wishes,

Phil Despain

Quick Tips

If you are eating at a place not in this book try using these quick tips to stay on track of your fitness goals and enjoy your meal.

1. Always pick grilled foods instead of fried.

2. Always choose poultry or fish over red meat.

3. Always pick veggies for your sides.

4. Always ask for your sauces and dressings on the side.

5. When you are having a salad always use a fat free dressing.

6. Choose to drink water and drink a full glass before your meal.

7. Never order an appetizer or dessert.

8. When you are unsure about the calories in a meal split the meal with someone or ask the waiter/waitress for a box with your food and place half the meal in the box.

Applebees

Fo od	Cal	Protein	Carbs	Fat
7oz House Sirloin, Ball Tip without sides	200	38g	1g	5g
9oz House Sirloin, Ball Tip without sides	270	49g	2g	7g
Napa Chicken & Portobello's	500	50g	38g	16g
Pepper-Crusted Sirloin & Whole Grains	350	28g	41g	10g
Thai Shrimp Salad	390	23g	32g	19g
Blackened Tilapia	450	31g	45g	17g
Chicken Noodle Soup - Lunch	120	9g	13g	3.5g
House Salad Lunch with Fat Free Italian Dressing	135	6g	12g	7g
Sides	**Cal**	**Protein**	**Carbs**	**Fat**
Seasonal Vegetables	35-60	1-5g	7-11g	0-.5g
Phil's Choice	**Cal**	**Protein**	**Carbs**	**Fat**
7oz House Sirloin, Ball Tip with Seasonal Vegetables	235-260	39-43g	8-12g	5-5.5g

Arbys

Food	Cal	Protein	Carbs	Fat
Classic Roast Beef Sandwich	255	19g	17.5g	12g
Jr. Ham & Cheddar Sandwich	210	14g	25g	6g
Grand Turkey Club (no mayo or bacon)	310	24g	36g	8g
Jr. Turkey & Cheese Sandwich	220	17g	23g	6g
Roast Turkey Farmhouse Salad with Light Italian Dressing (no cheese)	140	16g	9g	4.5g
Sides	**Cal**	**Protein**	**Carbs**	**Fat**
Chopped Side Salad	70	5g	4g	5g
Phil's Choice	**Cal**	**Protein**	**Carbs**	**Fat**
Jr. Turkey &Cheese Sandwich with Chopped Side Salad	290	22g	27g	11g

Burger King

Food	Cal	Protein	Carbs	Fat
Bacon Cheeseburger Deluxe on ½ bun (no cheese)	190	8g	16.5g	9g
Cheeseburger on ½ bun (no cheese)	170	7g	14.5g	8g
Tendergrill Chicken Sandwich on ½ bun	260	23g	24g	7.75g
Whopper Jr. on ½ bun	170	7g	15.5g	8g
Chicken, Apple & Cranberry Salad (no blue-cheese)	270	25g	35g	4g
Chicken Caesar Salad	270	32g	16g	9g
Breakfast	**Cal**	**Protein**	**Carbs**	**Fat**
Bacon, Egg Croisson'wich	225	9g	15.5g	13.5g
Ham, Egg Croisson'wich	235	13g	17.5g	12.5g
Original Maple Flavored Oatmeal	170	4g	32g	19g
Sides	**Cal**	**Protein**	**Carbs**	**Fat**
Apple Slices	30	0g	7g	0g
Phil's Choice	**Cal**	**Protein**	**Carbs**	**Fat**
Tendergrill Chicken Sandwich on ½ bun with Apple Slices	290	23g	31g	7.75g

Café Rio

Food	Cal	Protein	Carbs	Fat
6" Corn Tortilla	70	1g	13g	1g
Black Beans	140	8g	21g	2g
Pinto Beans	150	8g	23g	2.5g
Fire Grilled Chicken	100	17g	1g	2g
Mahi Mahi	70	13g	<1g	.05g
Fire Grilled Salmon	90	14g	<1g	2.5g
Lettuce	5	0g	<1g	0g
Sauce	**Cal**	**Protein**	**Carbs**	**Fat**
Tomatillo Sauce	30	1g	4g	1g
Red Chili Sauce	40	1g	5g	2g
Phil's Choice	**Cal**	**Protein**	**Carbs**	**Fat**
6"Corn Tortilla, Black Beans, Fire Grilled Chicken, Lettuce, Tomatillo Sauce	345	27g	39g	6g

Carls Jr.

Food	Cal	Protein	Carbs	Fat
Original Grilled Chicken Salad	280	18g	26g	12g
Redhook Beer Battered Cod Fish Sandwich on ½ bun	425	17g	50g	17.5
Charbroiled Chicken Club on ½ bun (no mayo)	400	33g	45g	14g
Charbroiled Santa Fe Chicken Sandwich (no sauce, no cheese)	430	30g	45g	14g
Charbroiled BBQ Chicken Sandwich	390	30g	50g	7g
Side	Cal	Protein	Carbs	Fat
Garden Side Salad	110	4g	14g	4.5g
Dressing	Cal	Protein	Carbs	Fat
Low Fat Balsamic Dressing	35	0g	5g	1.5g
Phil's Choice	Cal	Protein	Carbs	Fat
Original Grilled Chicken Salad with Low Fat Balsamic Dressing	315	18g	31g	13.5g

Chick-fil-A

Food	Cal	Protein	Carbs	Fat
Chick-fil-A Grilled Chicken Sandwich	320	30g	40g	5g
Grilled Nuggets 8 count	140	23g	4g	3g
Grilled Nuggets 12 count	200	34g	6g	4.5g
Grilled Market Salad	200	23g	17g	5g
Hearty Breast of Chicken Soup Medium	140	12g	18g	3g
Breakfast	Cal	Protein	Carbs	Fat
Plain Multigrain Oatmeal	140	0g	28g	3g
Sides	Cal	Protein	Carbs	Fat
Side Salad	80	5g	6g	5g
Phil's Choice	Cal	Protein	Carbs	Fat
Grilled Nuggets 12 Count and Side Salad	280	39g	12g	9.5g

Chilis

Food	Cal	Protein	Carbs	Fat
South West Chicken Soup- Cup	110	4g	13g	5g
Lunch Combo Fresco Salad	70	2g	4g	5g
6oz Sirloin with Grilled Avocado	410	39g	21g	20g
6oz Classic Sirloin	300	34g	1g	18g
Margarita Grilled Chicken	190	31g	8g	4g
Ancho Salmon	420	42g	7g	25g
Sides	**Cal**	**Protein**	**Carbs**	**Fat**
Spinach & Garlic Roasted Tomatoes	45	3g	9g	0g
Steamed Broccoli	40	3g	8g	0g
Phil's Choice	**Cal**	**Protein**	**Carbs**	**Fat**
Margarita Grilled Chicken with Steamed Broccoli	230	34g	16g	4g

Costa Vida

Food	Cal	Protein	Carbs	Fat
Quesadilla (black beans, corn tortilla, salsa fresca, shredded chicken)	257	32g	26g	2.2g
Small Mango Chicken Salad (shredded chicken, black beans, mango dressing)	308	17g	23g	16g
Phil's Choice	Cal	Protein	Carbs	Fat
Quesadilla (black beans, corn tortilla, salsa fresca, shredded chicken)	257	32g	26g	2.2g

IHOP

Food	Cal	Protein	Carbs	Fat
3 Original Buttermilk Pancakes	410	12g	60g	14g
Simple & Fit 2 – Egg Breakfast	350	25g	44g	9g
Simple & Fit Vegetable Omelette	310	27g	27g	12g
Mixed Greens House Salad with Fat Free Raspberry Vinaigrette	80	1g	17g	0g
Simple & Fit Mixed Greens House Salad with Reduced Fat Italian	40	2g	6g	1.5g
Plain Baked Potato	340	7g	63g	7g
Sides	**Cal**	**Protein**	**Carbs**	**Fat**
Seasonal Mixed Fruit	60	1g	17g	0g
Phil's Choice	**Cal**	**Protein**	**Carbs**	**Fat**
Simple & Fit Vegetable Omelette	310	27g	27g	12g

Kentucky Fried Chicken

Food	Cal	Protein	Carbs	Fat
Kentucky Grilled Chicken1Drumstick	90	13g	0g	4g
Chicken Little on ½ bun (no mayo)	165	12.5g	14.5g	7.5g
Crispy Chicken BLT Salad with Light Italian Dressing (no chicken)	110	9g	9g	5g
Crispy Chicken Caesar Salad with Light Italian Dressing (no chicken)	90	7g	7g	4.5g
Sides	Cal	Protein	Carbs	Fat
Corn on the Cob	70	2g	16g	.5g
Green Beans	25	1g	4g	0g
House Side Salad with Light Italian Dressing	30	1g	5g	.5g
Caesar Side Salad with Light Italian Dressing	40	3g	2g	2g
Phil's Choice	Cal	Protein	Carbs	Fat
Kentucky Grilled Chicken 2 Drumsticks and Green Beans	205	27g	4g	8g

McDonalds

Food	Cal	Protein	Carbs	Fat
Cheeseburger on ½ bun	215	12g	19g	10g
Hamburger on ½ bun	165	10g	18g	7g
Premium Bacon Ranch Salad with Low Fat Balsamic Vinaigrette (no chicken)	180	10g	15g	10g
Premium Bacon Ranch Salad with Grilled Chicken and Low Fat Balsamic Vinaigrette	300	34g	15g	11g
Premium South West Salad (no chicken no dressing)	230	8g	28g	10g
Premium South West Salad with Grilled Chicken (no dressing)	340	32g	28g	11g
Artisan Grilled Chicken Sandwich on ½ bun	250	28g	22.5g	5g
Breakfast	**Cal**	**Protein**	**Carbs**	**Fat**
Fruit and Yogurt Parfait	150	4g	30g	2g
Fruit and Maple Oatmeal (without brown sugar)	260	5g	49g	4g
Egg White Delight McMuffin	250	18g	30g	8g
Sides	**Cal**	**Protein**	**Carbs**	**Fat**
Side Salad with Balsamic Vinaigrette	50	1g	7g	2.5g
Apple Slices	15	0g	4g	0g
Yoplait Go-gurt	50	2g	9g	.5g
Phil's Choice	**Cal**	**Protein**	**Carbs**	**Fat**
Premium Bacon Ranch Salad with Grilled Chick, Low Fat Balsamic Vinaigrette and Apple Slices	315	34g	19g	11g

Olive Garden

Food	Cal	Protein	Carbs	Fat
Baked Tilapia with Shrimp	360	52g	12g	12g
Herb-Grilled Salmon	460	43g	8g	28g
Garlic Rosemary Chicken	540	62g	30g	20g
Citrus Chicken Sorrento	550	58g	36g	21g
Garden Primavera	560	16g	70g	25g
Grilled Chicken Caesar Salad	390	40g	12g	20g
Famous House Salad & Dressing (no croutons)	110	1g	6g	9g
Phil's Choice	Cal	Protein	Carbs	Fat
Garlic Rosemary Chicken	540	62g	30g	20g

Panda Express

Food	Cal	Protein	Carbs	Fat
Mixed Veggies	80	4g	16g	.5g
Mushroom Chicken	170	12g	11g	9g
String Bean Chicken Breast	190	14g	13g	9g
Broccoli Beef	150	9g	13g	7g
Phil's Choice	Cal	Protein	Carbs	Fat
Mixed Veggies with Broccoli Beef	230	13g	29g	7.5g

Red Lobster

Food	Cal	Protein	Carbs	Fat
Snow Crab Legs 1lbs (includes corn and potatoes)	370	46g	35g	5g
Live Main Lobster (includes corn and potatoes)	420	60g	35g	5g
Parmesan Crusted Tilapia	370	39g	17g	16g
Maple Glazed Chicken Dinner	500	54g	52g	8g
Sailor's Platter	320	46g	6g	10g
Flounder/Sole (oven broiled)	220	33g	7g	4.5g
Blackened Farm Raised Catfish	220	37g	0	8g
Golden Fried Farm Raised Catfish	230	31g	3g	10g
Garlic Shrimp Scampi	100	13g	1g	4.5g
Cod	200	36g	8g	2.5g
Fresh Flounder	250	39g	7g	5g
Grouper	240	48g	7g	2g
Halibut	230	43g	9g	2.5g
Perch	180	34g	8g	1.5g
Fresh Sole	190	37g	7g	2g
Pacific Snapper	210	36g	9g	3g
Sides	**Cal**	**Protein**	**Carbs**	**Fat**
Broccoli	50	4g	7g	.5g
Petite Green Beans	90	2g	8g	6g
Asparagus (seasonal)	60	3g	5g	3.5g
Phil's Choice	**Cal**	**Protein**	**Carbs**	**Fat**
Maple Glazed Chicken Dinner	500	54g	52g	8g

Red Robin

Food	Cal	Protein	Carbs	Fat
Simply Grilled Chicken Burger lettuce wrap (no margarine)	115	19g	8g	2g
Teriyaki Chicken Burger lettuce wrap (no mayo, no margarine)	342	30g	39g	10g
California Chicken Burger lettuce wrap (no bacon, no margarine)	230	25g	7g	13g
Whiskey River BBQ Chicken Burger lettuce wrap (no mayo, no margarine, no onion straws)	255	27g	17g	9g
Simply Grilled Chicken Salad (no croutons, no garlic bread)	260	31g	13g	11g
Sides	Cal	Protein	Carbs	Fat
Steamed Broccoli	32	3g	6g	0g
South West Black Beans	74	4g	15g	0g
Phil's Choice	Cal	Protein	Carbs	Fat
Teriyaki Chicken Burger lettuce wrap and Steamed Broccoli	374	33g	45g	10g

Ruby Tuesday

Food	Cal	Protein	Carbs	Fat
Petite Sirloin	355	35g	11g	19g
Hickory Bourbon Chicken	355	41g	25g	10g
Petite Sliced Sirloin	379	27g	23g	20g
Hickory Bourbon Salmon	390	42g	16g	18g
Grilled Salmon	330	42g	0g	18g
Jumbo Skewered Shrimp	274	27g	0g	15g
Blackened Tilapia	200	32g	2g	7g
Chicken Bella	332	42g	7g	15g
Sides	**Cal**	**Protein**	**Carbs**	**Fat**
Fresh Grilled Zucchini	41	1g	4g	2g
Fresh Green Beans	68	1g	5g	4g
Fresh Steamed Broccoli	52	3g	7g	2g
Roasted Spaghetti Squash	54	1g	6g	3g
Fresh Grilled Asparagus	70	4g	8g	3g
Phil's Choice	**Cal**	**Protein**	**Carbs**	**Fat**
Hickory Bourbon Chicken and Grilled Zucchini	396	42g	29g	12g

Subway

Bread 6 Inches	Cal	Protein	Carbs	Fat
9 Grain Wheat	210	8g	40g	2g
Flatbread	220	7g	38g	4.5g
Multigrain Flatbread	220	7g	39g	4.5g
Sour Dough	210	8g	41g	3g
Sauces	**Cal**	**Protein**	**Carbs**	**Fat**
Fat Fee Honey Mustard	30	0g	7g	0g
Guacamole	70	1g	3g	6g
Light Mayo	50	0g	1g	5g
Mustard, Yellow & Deli Brown	5	0g	1g	0g
Olive Oil	45	0g	0g	5g
Subway Vinaigrette	50	0g	2g	5g
Vinegar	0	0g	0g	0g
Vegetable	**Cal**	**Protein**	**Carbs**	**Fat**
Avocado	60	1g	3g	5g
Tomato	5	0g	1g	0g
The Rest of the Veggies are 0 cal according to Subways serving sizes	0	0g	0g	0g
Meat 6 Inches	**Cal**	**Protein**	**Carbs**	**Fat**
Black Forest Ham	60	9g	3g	2g
Turkey Breast	60	9g	3g	1.5g
Oven Roasted Chicken Breast	90	14g	4g	2.5g
Roast Beef	90	15g	2g	2.5g

Taco Bell

Food	Cal	Protein	Carbs	Fat
Beefy Mini Quesadilla (no sauce)	180	9g	17g	9g
Cheese Roll Up	180	9g	15g	9g
Shredded Chicken Mini Quesadilla (no chipotle sauce)	150	12g	15g	5g
Fresco Crunchy Taco – Beef	150	6g	13g	8g
Fresco Soft Taco – Shredded Chicken	140	10g	16g	3.5g
Fresco Soft Taco – Steak	150	12g	16g	4g
Sides	Cal	Protein	Carbs	Fat
Black Beans and Rice	180	6g	30g	4g
Breakfast	Cal	Protein	Carbs	Fat
Sausage Flatbread Melt	300	11g	27g	17g
Phil's Choice	Cal	Protein	Carbs	Fat
Fresco Soft Taco – Shredded Chicken	140	10g	16g	3.5g

Texas Roadhouse

Food	Cal	Protein	Carbs	Fat
House Salad	248	Na	Na	Na
6oz Sirloin Steak	200	Na	Na	Na
Grilled BBQ Chicken	250	Na	Na	Na
Sides	Cal	Protein	Carbs	Fat
Sweet Potato (not loaded)	230	Na	Na	Na
Apple Sauce	100	Na	Na	Na
Fresh Vegetables	100	Na	Na	Na
Green Beans	100	Na	Na	Na
Phil's Choice	Cal	Protein	Carbs	Fat
Grilled BBQ Chicken with Fresh Vegetables	350	Na	Na	Na

TGI Fridays

Food	Cal	Protein	Carbs	Fat
Sizzling Sirloin & Spinach	410	49g	11g	19g
Sizzling Chicken & Spinach	410	50g	18g	15g
Lunch Grilled Chicken Cobb Salad with low fat balsamic vinaigrette	370	24g	19g	24g
Lunch Balsamic Glazed Chicken Caesar Salad	350	19g	19g	22g
Soup of the Day- Chicken Noodle	250	15g	33g	7g
Soup of the Day- Tortilla	210	14g	18g	10g
6 oz. Sirloin	330	38g	2g	19g
Jack Daniels Mixed Grill (6oz sirloin and chicken)	490	68g	28g	11.5
Sides	**Cal**	**Protein**	**Carbs**	**Fat**
Side of Fresh Broccoli	50	3g	10g	.5g
Phil's Choice	**Cal**	**Protein**	**Carbs**	**Fat**
Jack Daniels Mixed (6oz sirloin and chicken) Side of Fresh Broccoli	540	71g	38g	12g

Wendys

Food	Cal	Protein	Carbs	Fat
Strawberry Field Chicken Salad Full Size ½ dressing apple balsamic vinaigrette (no cheese)	350	34g	25g	13.5g
Asian Cashew Chicken Salad Full Size ½ dressing light spicy Asian	335	3.5g	25.5g	11.5g
BBQ Ranch Chicken Salad Full Size ½ dressing light spicy asian chili vinaigrette (no cheese)	395	39g	25.5g	15g
Apple Pecan Chicken Salad Full Size ½ dressing pomegranate vinaigrette (no cheese)	400	30g	43g	11g
Dave's Hot'N Juicy ¼ lbs ½ bun (no mayo, no cheese)	355	22.5g	22g	17g
Jr. Hamburger ½ bun	180	11g	13.5g	7.25g
Ultimate Chicken Grill ½ bun	275	30.5g	24g	6g
Grilled Chicken Wrap	260	19g	25g	10g
Sides	**Cal**	**Protein**	**Carbs**	**Fat**
Apple Slices	40	0g	9g	0g
Phil's Choice	**Cal**	**Protein**	**Carbs**	**Fat**
Ultimate Chicken Grill ½ bun and Apple Slices	315	30.5g	33g	6g

References

www.bk.com/menu

www.tacobell.com/nutrition/calculator

www.kfc.com/nutrition

www.chick-fil-a.com/food/meal

www.arbys.com/build-a-meal

www.applebees.com/~/media/docs/applebees_Nutritio
nal_Info.pdf

www.media.olivegarden.com/en_us/pdf/olive_garden
_nutrition.pdf

www.tgifridays.com/nutrition.pdf

www.redlobster.com/heath/nutrition/nutrition_facts.
pdf

www.ihop.com/-
/media/ihop/PDFs/nutritionalinformation.ashx

www.carlsjr.com/menu/nutritional_calculator

www.caferio.com/nutritional-new

www.pandaexpress.com/nutritionCalculator#/?plate=
twoentree

www.texasroadhouse.com/menu/intractive-menu

www.rubytuesday.com/assets/menu/pdf/informationa
l/nutrition_pdf

www.redrobin/customizer_hub#_customize

http://www.costavida.net/menu/

https://www.wendys.com/en-us/nutrition-info

References Continued

http://www.subway.com/menu/Product.aspx?CC=USA&LC=ENG&ProductId=5&MenuId=35&MenuTypeId=1

http://www.mcdonalds.com/us/en/food/full_menu/full_menu_explorer.html

http://www.chilis.com/EN/Pages/menu.aspx